Married Women Weight Loss Fix

A Doctor's Guide to Regaining Confidence, Energy, and Health after Marriage

AF657955

Author: Dr. Amaresan Selvam

Published By

True Dreamster Press

ISBN: 978-93-6288-225-7

MRP: Rs.299/-

Printed in India

Dedication

To my beloved son, **Magizhnan**
You are my light, my strength, and my constant reminder that true health is the greatest wealth. Every word in this book carries a piece of my love for you.

To my dearest parents, **Appa and Amma**
Your unconditional love, sacrifices, and unwavering support have been the roots of all my achievements. This journey belongs to you as much as it does to me.

To my respected professor, **Dr. Narmada Ma'am**
Who first awakened in me the joy of reading and the power of books. Your inspiration shaped the path I walk today.

To my mentor, **Dr. Punnagai**
Whose wisdom, kindness, and encouragement guided me through my postgraduate journey and beyond.

This book is not mine alone—it is yours, as much as it is mine.

Author's Note

Being a family physician for more than 15 years, I have met countless women who walk into my clinic with a silent burden on their shoulders. Behind the smile, they show the world, many struggle with weight gain after marriage—whether due to pregnancies, hormonal changes, stress, or the endless responsibilities of managing both home and career.

I have seen the frustration in their eyes when the weighing scale doesn't move, the guilt when they compare themselves to their younger selves, and the sadness when society's unrealistic standards make them feel "less than." Many of these women are not just battling extra kilos—they are battling depression, fatigue, low self-confidence, and a loss of identity.

This book was born from those stories. It is not about quick fixes or crash diets. It is about **understanding your body, respecting your journey, and rebuilding your health with science, compassion, and practical steps.**

I wrote this book for every married woman who has ever stood in front of a mirror and wished for her old self-back. You are not alone, and you don't have to suffer in silence. With the right knowledge and small, consistent changes, you can reclaim your energy, confidence, and joy.

This is my heartfelt attempt to give you tools that actually work—not just for weight loss, but for a happier, healthier life.

With care and respect,
Dr. Amaresan Selvam, MD
Family Physician

Table of Contents

Introduction

"The Married Woman's Fat Loss Fix"

Introduction – A New Beginning

Marriage is often celebrated as the start of a beautiful journey — a life shared with love, responsibilities, and dreams. But for many women, marriage also quietly marks the beginning of an unexpected struggle: weight gain.

In the first few years of marriage, countless women notice their waistline expanding, their energy fading, and their confidence slipping. Some blame busy schedules, some point to hormonal changes, and others simply surrender, thinking, *"This is what happens after marriage."*

But here's the truth: **weight gain after marriage is not your destiny.**
It's not a punishment for love, nor a price you must pay for building a family. It's the result of subtle lifestyle changes, hormonal shifts, emotional stress, and societal patterns that no one talks about openly.

This book is not just another "diet guide." It is a **complete blueprint for married women** who want to take charge of their body, health, and confidence — without guilt, without confusion, and without falling for unsustainable fads.

Inside these pages, you will learn:

- Why women really gain weight after marriage (and why it's not your fault).
- How your hormones and metabolism influence fat storage.
- Simple nutrition and exercise strategies that actually work in a busy married life.
- The truth about intermittent fasting, supplements, and detox myths.
- How to rebuild your confidence, manage stress, and maintain results long term.

Most importantly, this book is about **power**.
Because when you lose weight the right way, you don't just look better — **you feel unstoppable.** You reclaim your energy, your happiness, and the freedom to live life on your terms.

So, whether you are newly married, a mother, or someone who has struggled for years, know this: **you are not alone, and you can take your power back.**

Welcome to your new beginning.

Your Weight Loss Journey at a Glance

Why Weight Gain Happens

It's not your fault!

Hormones & Metabolism

Influence on fat storage

Nutrition & Exercise

Strategies for married life

Intermittent Fasting & More

Supplements, detox myths

Confidence & Lasting Results

Rebuild body image, manage stres

A Quick Reality Check

You don't need to:

- Starve yourself.
- Workout 6days a week.
- Count every calorie.
- Cut carbs forever.

You do need:

- A structure that fits your life.
- A smarter way to eat and train.
- A mindset that isn't ruled by guilt.
- And a bit of self-compassion along the way.

This isn't just about weight loss. It's about reclaiming control. It's about showing up in your best form — physically, emotionally, hormonally — and doing so without burnout, guilt, or guessing games.

So, if you've been feeling stuck… or slowly fading behind the woman you used to be — take a breath. You've just opened the right book.

Your reset starts now.

Chapter 1

THE MARRIAGE WEIGHT TRAP – WHY WOMEN GAIN AFTER TYING THE KNOT

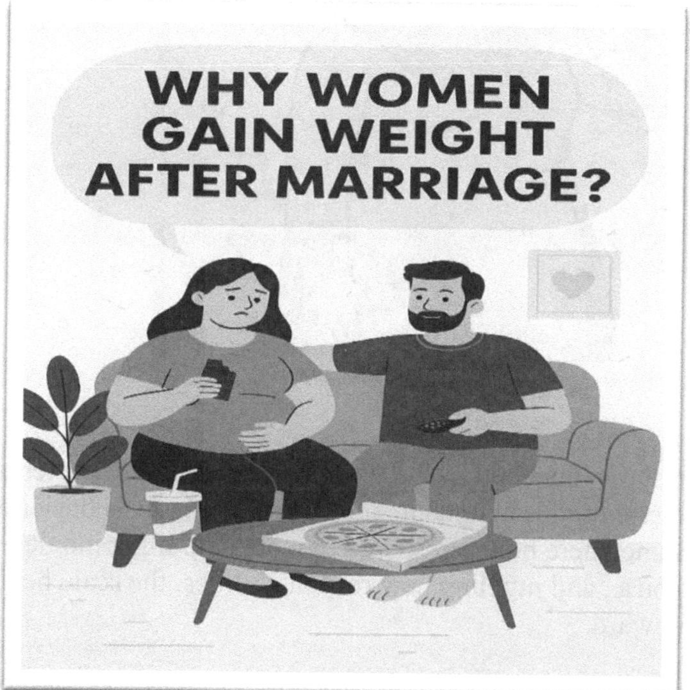

"It's not you. It's biology, routine—and real life."

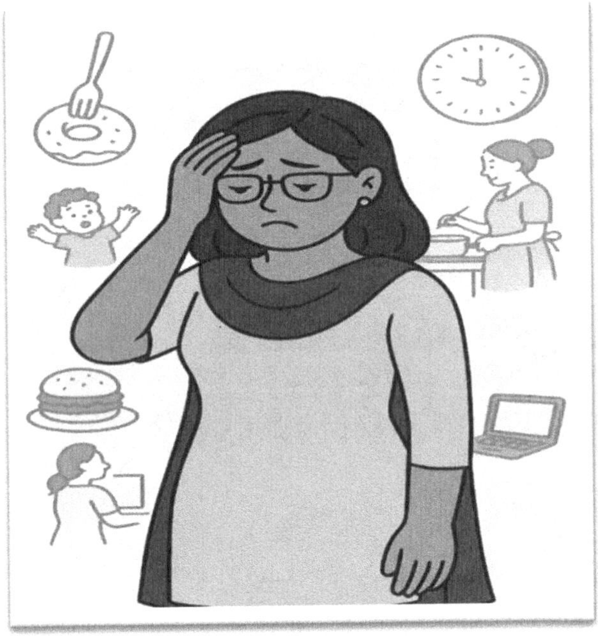

It often starts innocently. The wedding is over, family celebrations are endless, food is abundant, and life suddenly feels busier than ever. Somewhere between shared dinners, late-night movies with your spouse, and juggling new responsibilities, the scale begins to creep upward.

But why does this happen to so many women after marriage?

1. Lifestyle Shifts

Before marriage, many women follow routines centered around themselves — gym sessions, morning walks, or simple mindful eating. After marriage, routines change. Eating times are adjusted to the family, physical activity takes a backseat, and priorities shift. Slowly, calories consumed exceed calories burned.

2. Emotional & Social Eating

Marriage brings joy, but it also brings stress. Arguments, in-law expectations, or even simple household adjustments can create emotional turbulence. Food, especially comfort foods like sweets, fried snacks, or late-night munchies, becomes a coping mechanism. Add frequent family gatherings and festivals, and overeating feels unavoidable.

3. Hormonal Factors

Marriage often coincides with age-related hormonal changes. Rising insulin resistance, thyroid fluctuations, and in some cases PCOS, make fat storage easier and fat loss harder. Add contraceptive pills or stress-induced hormonal imbalances, and the weight gain feels sudden and stubborn.

4. Cultural Patterns

In many Indian households, love is expressed through food. A caring spouse may insist, *"Just one more chapati,"* or a mother-in-law may say, *"You look weak, eat more."* Refusing food feels disrespectful, and soon, guilt-free eating becomes guilt-laden overeating.

5. Sedentary Living

For many newly married women, professional and family responsibilities demand long sitting hours. With less movement and little time for structured exercise, metabolism slows, fat accumulates, and the body begins to change.

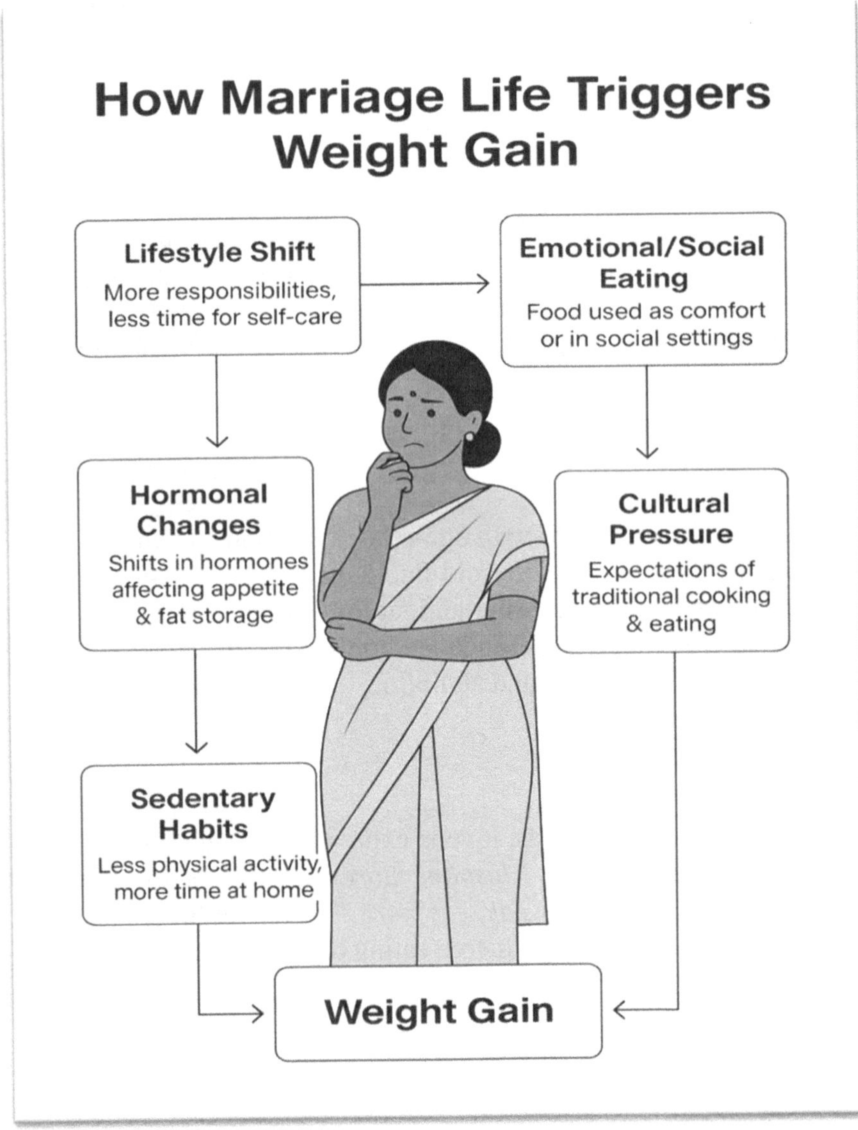
How Marriage Life Triggers Weight Gain
Lifestyle Shift
More responsibilities, less time for self-care
Emotional/Social Eating
Food used as comfort or in social settings
Hormonal Changes
Shifts in hormones affecting appetite & fat storage
Cultural Pressure
Expectations of traditional cooking & eating
Sedentary Habits
Less physical activity, more time at home
Weight Gain

🪜 The Good News: You're Not Broken

You didn't fail. You adapted. You responded to love, safety, and new roles. That means you can also adapt again — intentionally this time.

The goal of this book is not to shame your past, but to reshape your future — with science, structure, and sanity.

Chapter 2

HORMONES & BELLY FAT – THE SECRET CONNECTION

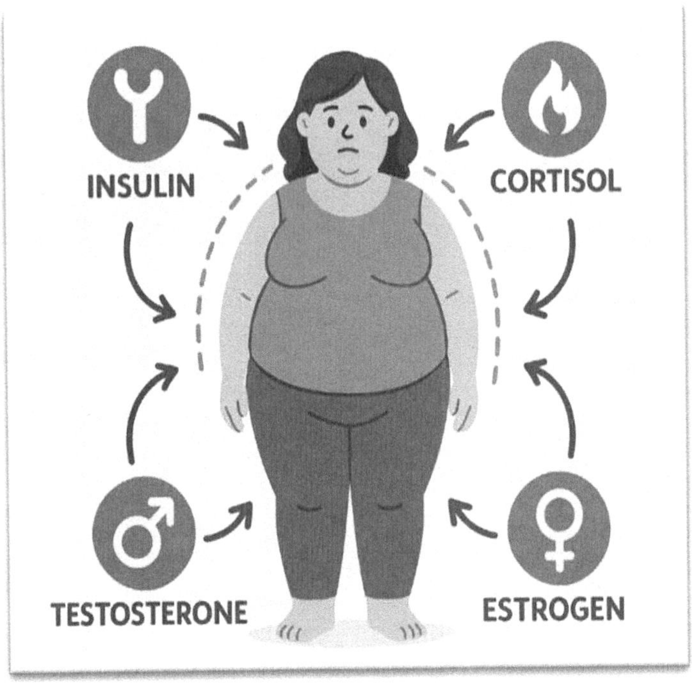

Fat loss isn't just calories in vs. calories out. It's chemistry, too.

When most women think about weight gain, the first explanation that comes to mind is simple: *"I must be eating too much and moving too little."*

But if weight was only about calories in and calories out, then every woman who dieted strictly would stay slim forever. Yet, the reality is different. Many married women find themselves gaining weight even when they eat less than before. Why? The answer lies in one powerful word: **hormones.**

Hormones are your body's **chemical messengers**. They control hunger, fat storage, metabolism, mood, and even where fat gets deposited on your body. When your hormones are balanced, fat loss feels natural. But when they are out of balance, weight gain can feel inevitable — no matter how disciplined you are.

Let's break down the main hormonal players that influence belly fat in married women:

1. Insulin – The Fat Storage Hormone

Insulin's job is to help your body use or store glucose from food. But in today's lifestyle — high-carbohydrate meals, frequent snacking, and late-night dinners — insulin levels are almost always elevated.

- High insulin = your body is constantly in "fat-storage mode."
- This makes it harder to burn fat, especially around the belly and thighs.

Marriage often means more frequent shared meals, desserts at family functions, and eating at odd times. This constant food availability keeps insulin high — and fat loss low.

2. Cortisol – The Stress Hormone

Marriage brings happiness, but also stress: managing relationships, household responsibilities, work-life balance, or parenting. Chronic stress triggers **cortisol**, which signals your body to store fat — particularly in the abdominal area.

That's why many women notice a "stress belly." Even if calories are controlled, high cortisol keeps the body holding on to fat.

3. Estrogen & Progesterone – The Female Balance

Hormonal fluctuations during different life phases — from contraceptive pills to pregnancy and perimenopause — all influence weight.

- Too much estrogen relative to progesterone can lead to fat storage in the hips and thighs.
- Low progesterone can cause bloating, mood swings, and sugar cravings.

This is why many women feel their body "changes shape" after marriage and childbirth, even if their weight on the scale hasn't dramatically increased.

4. Thyroid Hormones – The Metabolic Switch

The thyroid gland is your body's thermostat. If it slows down, metabolism slows too. For many women, subtle thyroid imbalances (common in India) go undiagnosed, leading to unexplained fatigue, hair fall, and stubborn weight gain.

Marriage and childbirth can sometimes trigger thyroid issues, making it crucial to test and treat early.

5 Key Hormones That Influence Fat

Hormone	Role	How It Affects Fat	How to Fix
Cortisol	Stress hormone	Increases during stress & lack of slep	Manage stress, improve sleep
Insulin ((storage hormone)	Insulines storage hormone	High levels cause fat gain, especially around organs	Limit sugary foods
Estrogen (Female hormone)	Peaks during menstrual cycles & pregnancy	Low estrogen causes body fat gain	Eat more fiber, cruciferous vegetables
Leptin (Satiety hormone)	Feel full & satisfied	Resistance leads to overeating & weight gain	Eat more protein
Ghrelin (Hunger	Feel hungry	High levels increase appetite & fat storage	Eat regularly, manage stress

5. Leptin & Ghrelin – The Hunger Hormones

Leptin tells your brain, *"You are full."* Ghrelin tells your brain, *"You are hungry."*

- Lack of sleep (common in married life, especially after kids) lowers leptin and raises ghrelin.
- The result? More hunger, more cravings, and more late night snacking.

Chapter 3

THE 5 METABOLIC MISTAKES MARRIED WOMEN MAKE

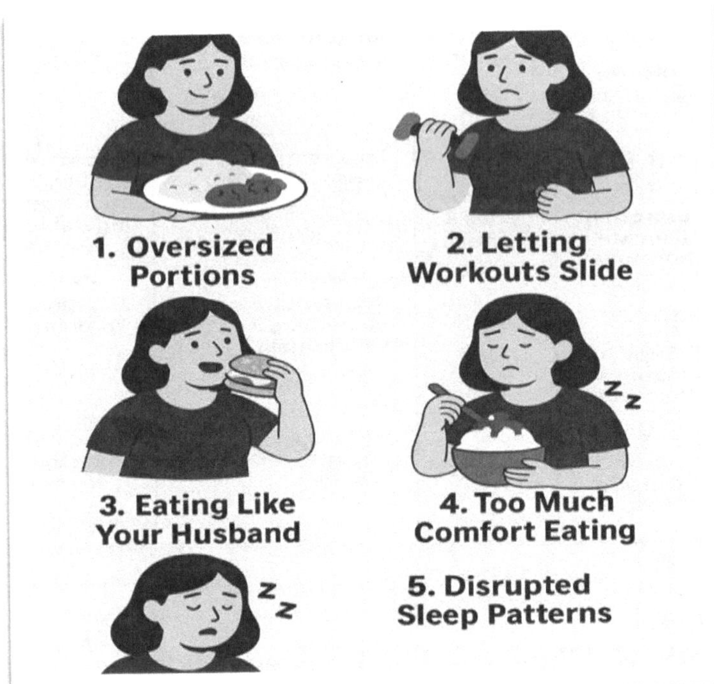
1. Oversized Portions
2. Letting Workouts Slide
3. Eating Like Your Husband
4. Too Much Comfort Eating
5. Disrupted Sleep Patterns

Most women don't realize that the little everyday choices they make after marriage slowly push their metabolism into a fat-storing mode. These not "big sins"— but small, repeated mistakes add up over months and years.

The good news? Once you recognize and correct them, your body can finally shift back into fat-burning mode.

Here are the **five most common metabolic mistakes married women make**:

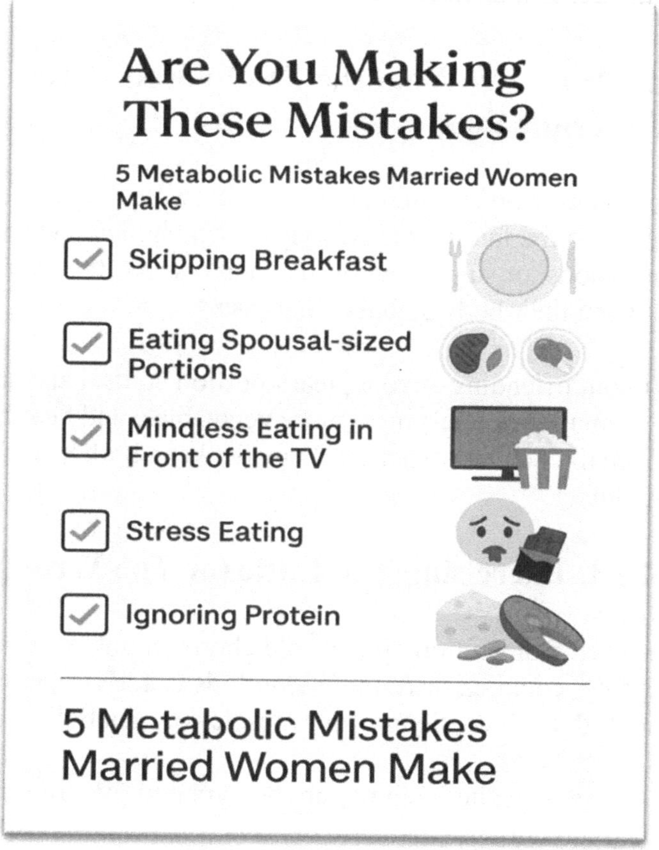
Are You Making These Mistakes?
5 Metabolic Mistakes Married Women Make
Skipping Breakfast
Eating Spousal-sized Portions
Mindless Eating in Front of the TV
Stress Eating
Ignoring Protein
5 Metabolic Mistakes Married Women Make

Mistake 1: Skipping Breakfast but Snacking All Day

Many women think skipping breakfast will save calories. But what usually happens?

- By mid-morning, hunger crashes in.
- Snacking on tea, biscuits, or sweets becomes routine.
- Insulin spikes throughout the day, locking the body in fat-storage mode.

Fix: If you prefer a late breakfast, that's fine (it's similar to intermittent fasting). But when you eat, make it **protein-rich** — eggs, paneer, sprouts, or dal — so cravings stay away.

Mistake 2: Eating What the Family Eats (Even When It Doesn't Suit You)

After marriage, women often give up their own eating preferences. They adjust to the family's food style — which may mean more rice, fried foods, or sugar. Out of love and respect, they keep eating it, even when their body signals otherwise.

Fix: Without offending anyone, learn portion control and subtle swaps — smaller rice servings, more vegetables, and healthier snacks. Small changes, consistently made, keep both health and harmony intact.

Mistake 3: Exercising Too Little (or Too Wrong)

Most married women think household chores count as exercise. But cleaning, cooking, or running after kids is **activity**, not **exercise**. It doesn't challenge your muscles or metabolism enough to burn fat.
Others do the opposite — they join the gym and overtrain for a few weeks, only to burn out and quit.

Fix: Aim for **simple, consistent workouts** — 20–30 minutes a day, mixing strength training (to boost metabolism) with walking or yoga (to calm the mind).

Mistake 4: Stress-Eating & Emotional Overeating

Marriage brings responsibilities: balancing work, family, children, finances, in-laws. Food becomes comfort. Stress eating is not a lack of willpower — it's your brain demanding quick dopamine through sugar and carbs.

Fix: Learn alternative stress relievers — journaling, a short walk, deep breathing, or even talking to a supportive friend. Replace emotional eating with emotional healing.

Mistake 5: Believing Quick Fixes & Diet Myths

"Detox juices will melt fat."
"Skipping dinner is the only way to slim down."
"Carbs are the enemy."
Sound familiar? Many married women jump from one fad to another — keto today, GM diet tomorrow, detox next week. The result? Short-term weight loss, followed by long-term frustration.

Fix: Stop chasing trends. Focus on **balanced nutrition, consistent activity, and hormonal health.** Sustainable fat loss is not about punishment — it's about building habits that last.

✅ ***Fix it:***

- Daily greens+fatty fish 2x/week.
- Consider a high-quality women's multi+magnesium glycinate.
- Get sunlight exposure daily, ideally before 10am.

↓ Final Thought:

You don’t need to be perfect —just precise.

Small, consistent shifts beat extreme programs every time. Fixing these five mistakes alone can jumpstart your metabolism and unlock steady, sustainable fat loss.

Chapter 4

THE FAT-LOSS NUTRITION PLAN THAT ACTUALLY WORKS

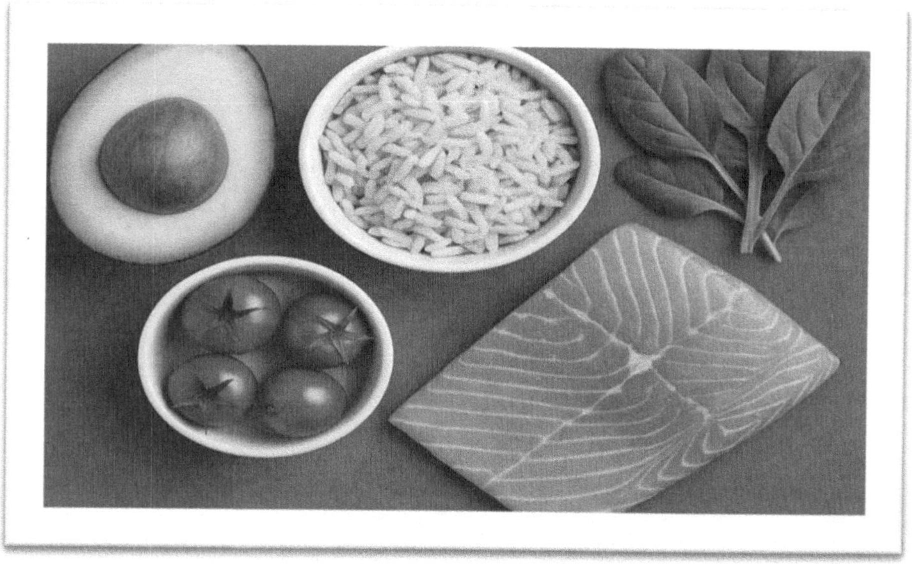

Most women think fat loss is about "eating less." But starving only slows down your metabolism and makes you crave more. The truth is simple: **you don't need to eat less — you need to eat right.**

A fat-loss plan should fit your life as a married woman — busy mornings, family meals, social functions, and unexpected cravings. That's why this plan is not about restrictions. It's about **smart food choices, portion control, and metabolic balance.**

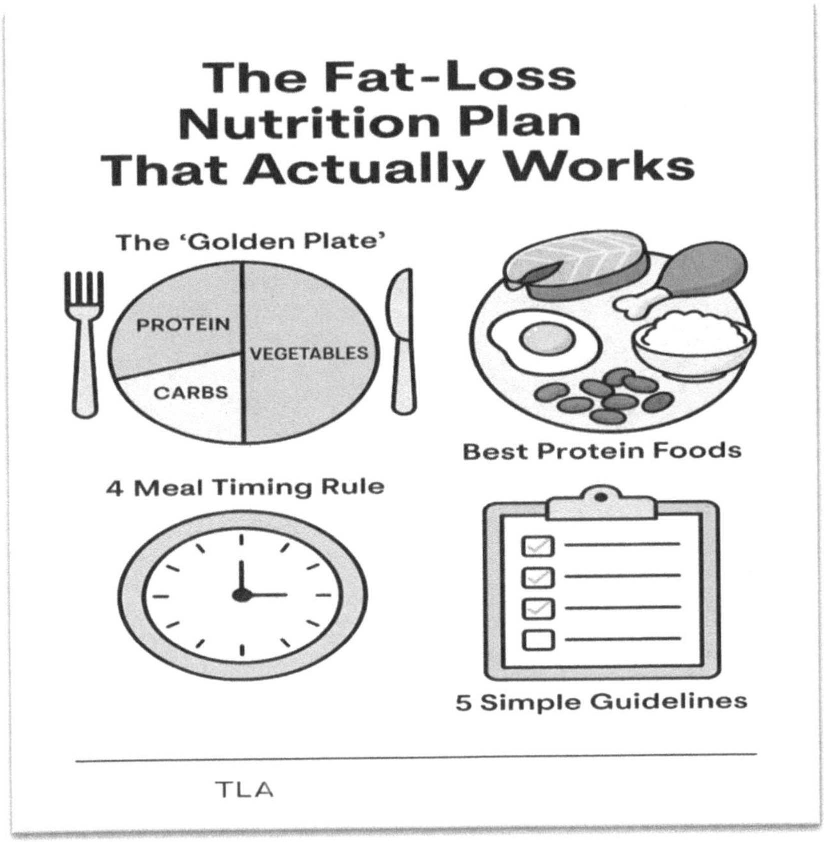

Here's your step-by-step guide:

Step 1: The Golden Plate Formula

Every meal should have:

- **½-plate vegetables** (cooked or raw) → fills you up, low in calories.
- **¼ plate protein** (dal, fish, chicken, eggs, paneer, and sprouts).
- **¼ plate carbs** (rice, chapati, millet, quinoa).

Why? This balances blood sugar, keeps insulin steady, and stops overeating.

Step 2: The 4 Meal Timing Rule

Instead of grazing all day, stick to **3 main meals + 1 light snack.**

- **Breakfast:** High in protein (e.g., 2 boiled eggs + vegetables OR paneer upma).
- **Lunch:** Balanced Indian thali (dal + sabji + 1–2 chapatis + salad).
- **Snack (4–5 pm):** Nuts + green tea OR fruit with peanut butter.
- **Dinner (by 8 pm):** Light and protein-rich (grilled fish, dal soup, paneer + salad).

Why? Frequent snacking keeps insulin high. Fewer, balanced meals give your body time to burn fat.

Step 3: The Protein Upgrade

Most Indian women eat plenty of carbs but very little protein. Low protein = muscle loss = slower metabolism.

- Aim for **60–70g protein/day** (spread across meals).

• Sources: dal, chana, paneer, eggs, chicken, fish, sprouts, soy, Greek yogurt.

Trick: With every meal, ask yourself: **"Where is my protein?"**

Step 4: Sugar & Oil – Cut Smart, Not Extreme

- Avoid sugary tea/coffee, juices, biscuits, packaged sweets.
- Switch to jaggery in small amounts, but not daily.
- Oils: stick to 2–3 tsp/day (groundnut, coconut, or ghee). Avoid deep-frying.

Remember: You don't need to ban foods — you need to **control frequency and portion.**

Step 5: Hydration & Mindful Eating

- Drink **2–3 liters water/day** (add lemon, jeera, or mint for flavor).
- Eat slowly, chew well. When you eat fast, you miss fullness signals and overeat.

Sample Indian-Friendly Day Plan

Morning (7 am): Warm water + lemon
Breakfast (8:30 am): 2 boiled eggs + spinach chapati OR paneer upma + green tea
Lunch (1 pm): 1 cup dal, 1 cup sabji, 1 chapati, ½ cup curd, salad
Snack (4:30 pm): A handful of almonds + 1 apple
Dinner (7:30 pm): Grilled chicken/fish OR paneer curry with sautéed vegetables
Bedtime (10 pm): Herbal tea (chamomile / jeera water)

✦ The Key Insight:

Fat loss is not about starving. It's about **fueling your body with the right foods, in the right portions, at the right time.** Once you master this formula, you'll feel energetic, satisfied, and in control.

Chapter 5

SMART EATING WITHOUT SPOUSAL RESISTANCE

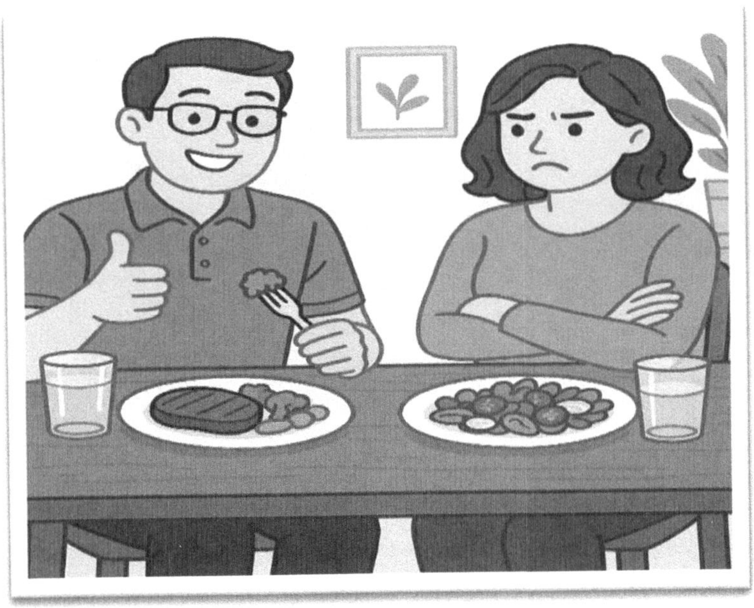

For many women, the real challenge is not *knowing* what to eat — it's being able to follow it at home without offending anyone. In Indian households, food is more than nutrition — it's an expression of love, culture, and family bonding.

So how do you stick to your fat-loss plan without creating fights, guilt, or unwanted pressure? Here are smart strategies that keep everyone happy while keeping your waistline safe.

1. The Art of Portion Diplomacy

You don't always have to say "No." Instead, say "Yes" — but in smaller amounts.

- When your spouse or in-laws insist, *"Have one more chapati"* → Take half instead of full.
- When sweets are served → Share one piece, or take a bite and save the rest for later.

Trick: Serve yourself in smaller plates. It looks full, but portions stay controlled.

2. Smart Food Swaps (That No One Notices)

Instead of rejecting traditional food, upgrade it quietly.

- Replace **refined atta** with multigrain or millet atta.
- Use **less oil** but add flavor with spices, herbs, and lemon.
- For dessert, make **fruit-based kheer** or baked alternatives.

Result: The family enjoys the same dish, but you eat healthier without anyone complaining.

3. The "Balance on Your Plate" Trick

If family meals are rice-heavy, don't argue. Just adjust your plate:

- Take a smaller serving of rice.
- Double your vegetables and dal.
- Add curd or salad to fill up.

This way, you eat what the family eats, but your metabolism stays balanced.

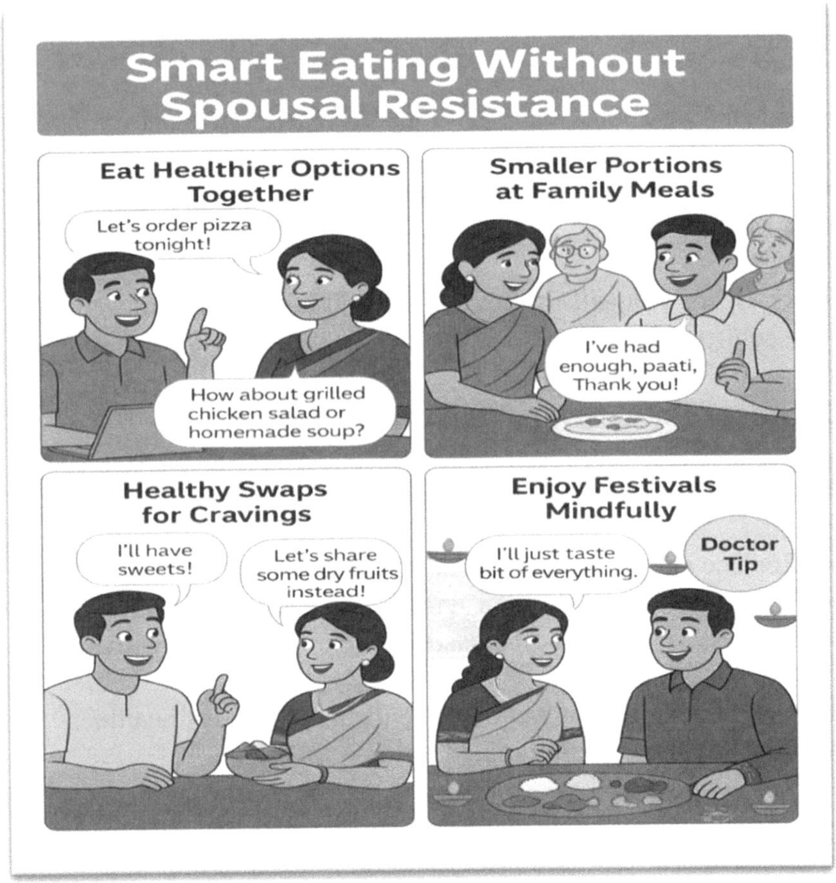
Smart Eating Without Spousal Resistance
Eat Healthier Options Together
Let's order pizza tonight!
How about grilled chicken salad or homemade soup?
Smaller Portions at Family Meals
I've had enough, paati, Thank you!
Healthy Swaps for Cravings
I'll have sweets!
Let's share some dry fruits instead!
Enjoy Festivals Mindfully
I'll just taste bit of everything.
Doctor Tip

4. Eat Before Functions & Gatherings

Family weddings, parties, or festivals are unavoidable. But you can control your choices.

- Eat a small protein snack (like boiled eggs or paneer) at home before going.
- At the event, enjoy small portions guilt-free without overindulging.

This way, you participate socially but protect your goals.

5. Communicate Without Conflict

Sometimes honesty is the best tool. Instead of saying, *"I'm dieting,"* try:

- *"I feel better with lighter food at night."*
- *"I'm focusing on my health — I want to be more energetic for all of us."*

Most spouses and families eventually respect and even admire these efforts when they see your energy improving.

🠗 The Key Insight:

Healthy eating after marriage doesn't mean rejecting family meals or traditions. It's about **quiet, smart strategies that allow you to enjoy love through food — without paying the price on your body.**

Bonus: Secretly Win Him Over

Once he sees you:

- Having more energy.
- Looking and feeling better.
- Not obsessing or depriving yourself.

He'll likely become curious and even follow your lead. Change often starts quietly — and leads loudly.

Chapter 6

THE MARRIED WOMAN'S WORKOUT RESET

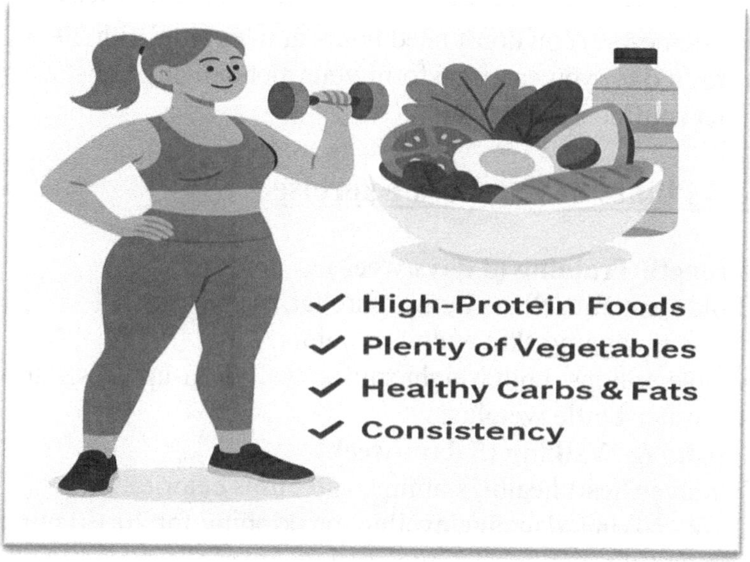
✓ High-Protein Foods
✓ Plenty of Vegetables
✓ Healthy Carbs & Fats
✓ Consistency

Most married women believe two things about exercise:

1. *"I don't have time."*
2. *"Housework is my workout."*

But here's the truth: **housework is activity, not exercise.** It keeps you moving, yes, but it doesn't challenge your muscles or metabolism enough to burn fat.

The good news? You don't need hours at the gym. With **20–30 minutes a day**, you can transform your metabolism, boost energy, and feel confident again.

The 3 Pillars of Fat-Loss Exercise

1. **Strength Training (3 days/week)**
- Builds lean muscle → burns more fat, even at rest.
- Prevents sagging skin and weak joints.
- Simple options: bodyweight squats, wall push-ups, resistance bands, water-bottle weights.

2. **Cardio & Walking (5 days/week)**
- Improves heart health, stamina, and burns calories.
- Brisk walking, dancing, cycling, or skipping for 20–30 minutes.
- Can be split into two 15-min sessions if time is short.

3. **Flexibility & Stress Relief (daily)**
- Yoga or stretching keeps the body agile and reduces stress hormones like cortisol.
- Just 10 minutes of breathing + stretches can calm your mind and prevent stress eating.

The 20-Minute Home Workout Plan

(No Equipment Needed)

Warm-up (2 min)

- March in place
- Arm rotations
- Neck + shoulder rolls

Workout (15 min)

- Squats – 15 reps
- Wall push-ups – 10 reps
- Step-ups on stairs – 20 steps
- Glute bridges – 12 reps
- Plank hold – 20–30 sec

(Repeat the circuit 2–3 times as per ability)

Cool-down (3 min)

- Stretch arms, legs, back
- Deep breathing (inhale 4 sec, exhale 6 sec)

Done! In less time than it takes to scroll Instagram, you've boosted your metabolism.

Lifestyle Movement Hacks

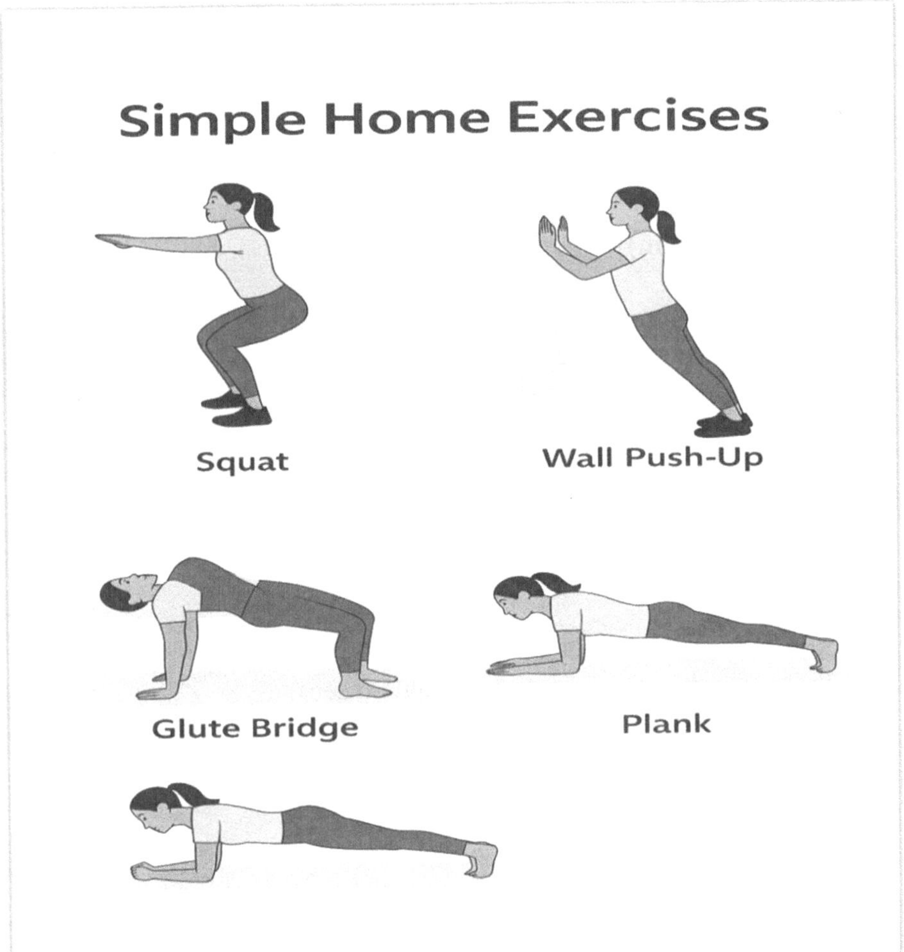

Even on days you can't "work out," keep moving:

- Take stairs instead of lift.
- Walk while talking on the phone.
- Play outdoor games with kids.
- Do "mini workouts" — 10 squats while waiting for tea, calf raises while brushing teeth.

✦ The Key Insight:

Exercise is not about punishing yourself. It's about building a body that supports your marriage, motherhood, career, and dreams. Just **20 minutes a day** can transform not only your body but your energy, mood, and confidence.

Chapter 7

SIMPLE HOME WORKOUTS FOR EVERY BODY

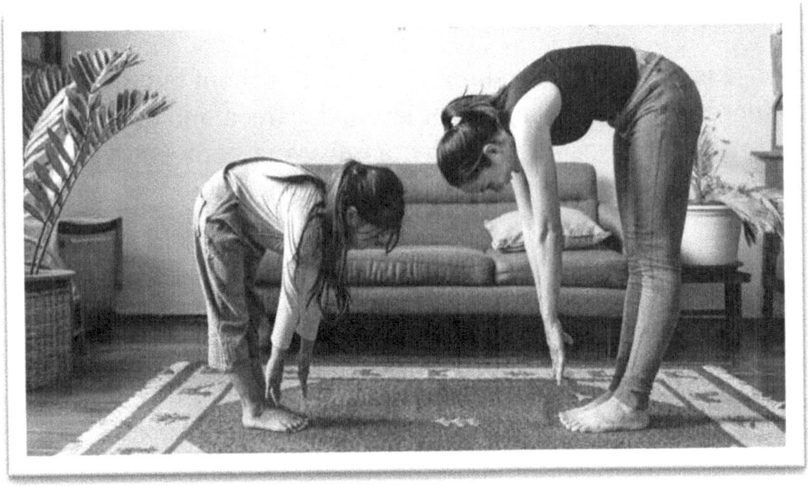

Not every woman starts from the same place. Some haven't exercised in years, some have back pain, while others may already walk regularly. That's why your workout plan should meet you where you are.

Here's a **step-by-step workout library**, designed for three levels: **Beginner → Intermediate → Advanced.**

Level 1: Beginner (For Women Who Haven't Exercised in Years)

Goal: Build stamina, confidence, and basic strength.
Duration: 15–20 minutes, 4 days/week

Warm-up (3 min)

- March in place
- Shoulder circles
- Neck rotations

Main Workout

- Wall Push-ups – 8–10 reps
- Chair Squats – 10 reps (sit and stand from chair)
- Standing Side Leg Lifts – 10 per side
- Cat-Cow Stretch – 5 reps
- Slow March – 1 min

Cool-down (2 min)

- Stretch arms overhead
- Gentle breathing

This is safe, easy, and perfect if you're starting from zero.

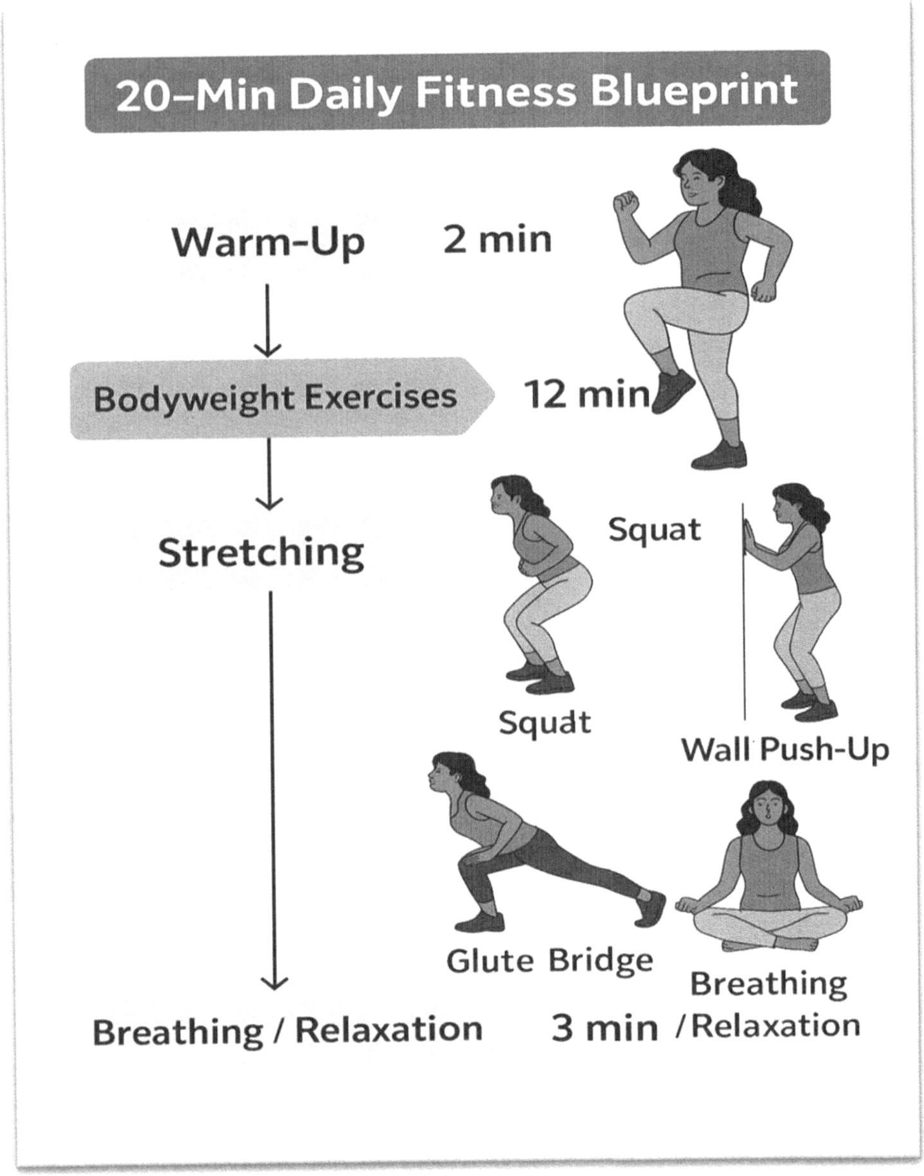
20-Min Daily Fitness Blueprint
Warm-Up
2 min
Bodyweight Exercises
12 min
Stretching
Squat
Squat
Wall Push-Up
Glute Bridge
Breathing /Relaxation
Breathing / Relaxation
3 min

Level 2: Intermediate (For Women Who Walk Regularly but Want More)

Goal: Burn fat, tone muscles, and improve energy.
Duration: 20–25 minutes, 4–5 days/week

Warm-up (3 min)

- Jumping jacks (or half-jacks if joint pain)
- Arm swings
- Hip rotations

Main Workout (Circuit, repeat 2–3 times)

- Squats – 12 reps
- Modified Push-ups (knees down) – 8–10 reps
- Step-ups (using stairs) – 20 steps
- Glute Bridges – 12 reps
- Plank Hold – 15–20 sec

Cool-down (3 min)

- Forward bend (touch toes softly)
- Deep breathing with hands on stomach

This stage starts shaping your body while boosting metabolism.

Level 3: Advanced (For Women Who Want to Push Themselves)

Goal: Maximum fat burn, strong core, toned body.
Duration: 25–30 minutes, 5–6 days/week

Warm-up (3 min)

- High knees – 30 sec
- Arm circles – 20 sec
- Shoulder shrugs – 20 sec

Main Workout (Circuit, repeat 3 times)

- Squats or Jump Squats – 15 reps
- Push-ups – 10 reps
- Burpees (or half-burpees if new) – 5 reps
- Mountain Climbers – 20 sec
- Side Plank – 20 sec each side

Cool-down (5 min)

- Cobra stretch
- Child's pose
- Gentle side stretch

This level will make you sweat — but it also sculpts your body and accelerates fat loss.

Bonus: The "Busy Day" 7-Minute Workout

For days when you truly don't have time:

- 20 Jumping Jacks
- 10 Squats
- 10 Push-ups (wall or floor)
- 20 Step-ups (stairs)
- 15 Glute Bridges
- 20-sec Plank

Done in 7 minutes — better than skipping!

The Key Insight:

No matter where you start, there's a workout for you. Consistency matters more than perfection. Whether it's **10 minutes of chair squats** or **30 minutes of advanced circuits**, every step brings you closer to your goal.

Chapter 8

THE 10-DAY RESET PLAN – KICKSTART YOUR TRANSFORMATION

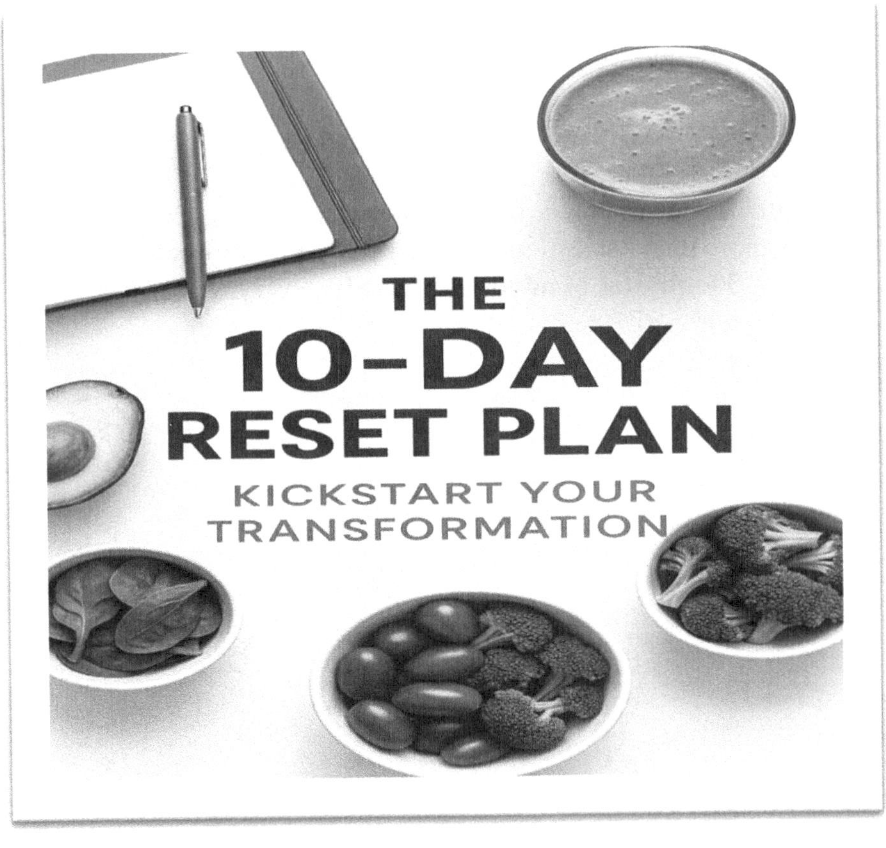

Sometimes, the hardest part of weight loss is just **getting started.** Married life is busy, routines are set, and the thought of a big lifestyle overhaul feels overwhelming.

That's why I created this **10-Day Reset Plan.**
It's not extreme. It's not about starving. It's about resetting your hormones, metabolism, and mindset so your body gets a **taste of fat-burning mode.**

In just 10 days, you will notice:
✅ Reduced bloating
✅ Better energy and focus
✅ Fewer cravings
✅ A jumpstart in fat loss

The 3 Golden Rules of the Reset

1. **No sugar, no junk, no alcohol** for 10 days (strict but short).
2. **3 meals + 1 snack only** (no all-day grazing).
3. **20 minutes movement daily** (workouts from Chapter 7).

The Daily Reset Routine

Morning (Start Your Day Right)

- Wake up: **Warm water with lemon** (kick-starts digestion).
- 10 min **stretching / yoga**.

Breakfast (High-Protein Start)

Options:

- 2 boiled eggs + sautéed vegetables
- Paneer bhurji + 1 millet roti
- Sprouts salad + buttermilk

Why? A protein-rich breakfast balances insulin and prevents cravings.

Midday Hydration

- 2–3 glasses of water
- Green tea / herbal tea (no sugar).

Lunch (Balanced Indian Plate)

- ½ plate vegetables (sabji/salad)
- ¼ plate protein (dal, chicken, fish, paneer)
- ¼ plate carbs (1 roti or ½ cup rice/millet)
- Curd (small bowl)

Why? Keeps energy steady without post-lunch crash.

Evening Snack (Light & Nutritious)

Options:

- A handful of almonds/walnuts
- 1 fruit (apple/guava) + herbal tea
- Roasted chana

Dinner (Light & Early – before 8 pm)

Options:

- Grilled fish or chicken + sautéed vegetables
- Paneer curry + salad
- Dal soup + steamed vegetables

Rule: Dinner must be lighter than lunch.

Night Routine

- 10 min **walk or stretching**.
- Warm jeera water or chamomile tea.
- Sleep by **10:30 pm** (crucial for fat loss).

Sample 10-Day Plan

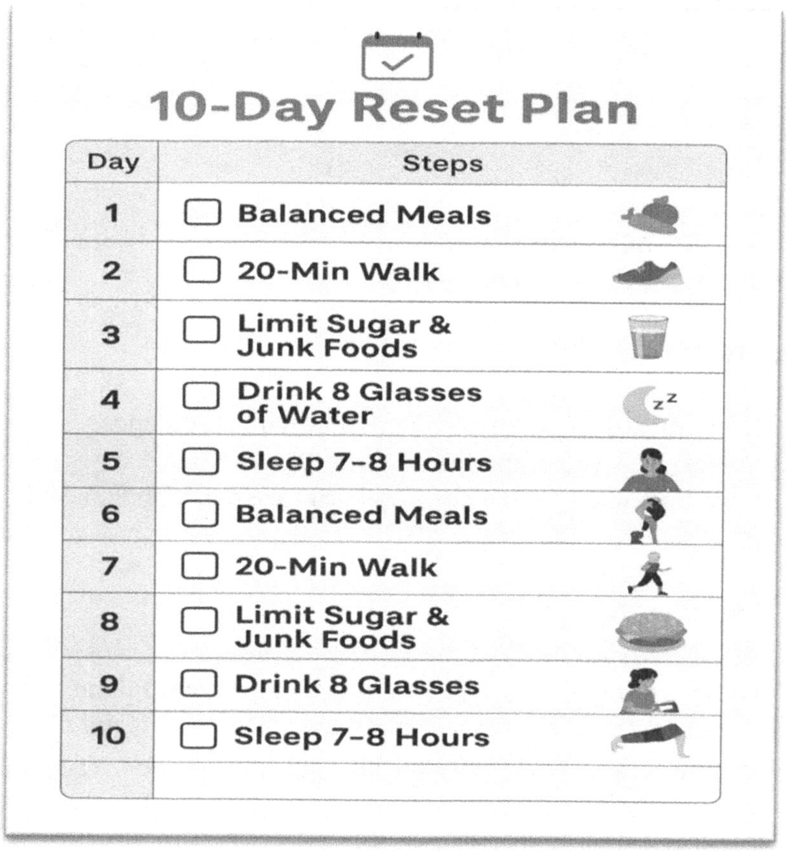

10-Day Reset Plan

Day	Steps
1	☐ Balanced Meals
2	☐ 20-Min Walk
3	☐ Limit Sugar & Junk Foods
4	☐ Drink 8 Glasses of Water
5	☐ Sleep 7–8 Hours
6	☐ Balanced Meals
7	☐ 20-Min Walk
8	☐ Limit Sugar & Junk Foods
9	☐ Drink 8 Glasses
10	☐ Sleep 7–8 Hours

Day 1–3:

- Follow meals strictly.
- 15 min Beginner Workout.
- No sugar, no fried food.

Day 4–6:

- Add Intermittent Fasting (12-hrs. gap between dinner & breakfast).
- 20 min Intermediate Workout.
- Notice cravings reducing.

Day 7–9:

- Stick to plan.
- Increase water intake.
- 25 min workout (add core exercises).

Day 10:

- Celebration day → not with junk, but with confidence.
- Reflect: You've completed 10 days of discipline.
- Reward yourself with a non-food gift (a saree, a book, a spa visit).

⏚ The Key Insight:

In 10 days, your body resets its **hormones and metabolism.** You'll feel lighter, more energetic, and motivated. The reset is not the destination — it's the **launch pad** for long-term fat loss.

Chapter 9

INTERMITTENT FASTING SIMPLIFIED

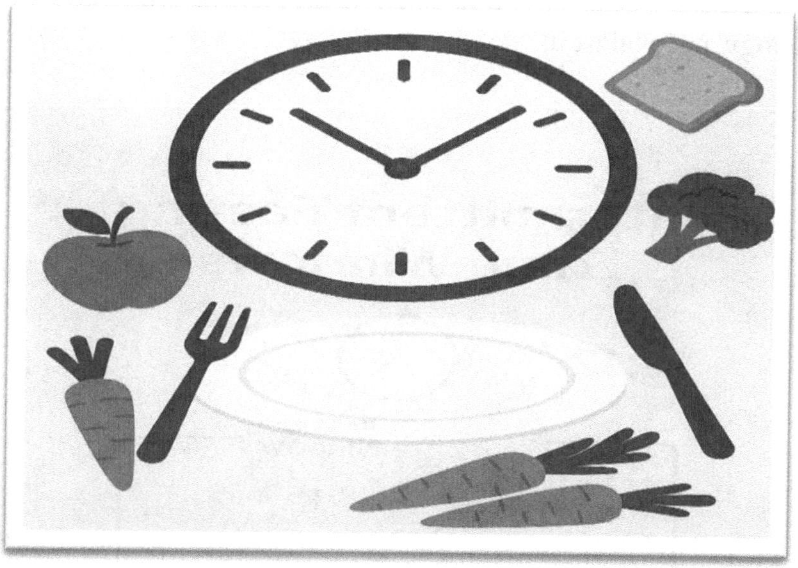

Intermittent Fasting (IF) is one of the most powerful, natural tools for fat loss — and it doesn't involve fancy diets, powders, or calorie counting.

It simply means: **eating during certain hours and giving your body a break from food during others.**

This break lowers insulin, improves fat-burning, and resets your metabolism. The beauty of IF is that it works with your body's biology, not against it.

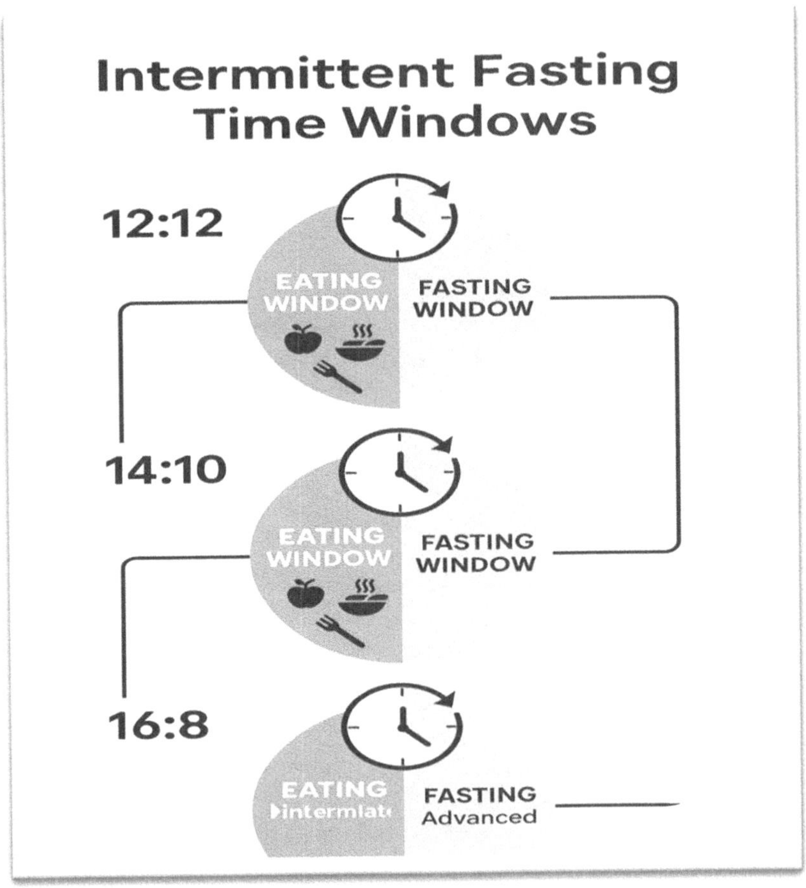

Why Intermittent Fasting Works

- **Insulin Reset:** When you stop eating every few hours, insulin levels drop, allowing your body to finally burn stored fat.
- **Fewer Cravings:** After a few days, hunger hormones stabilize. You feel less controlled by food.
- **Cellular Repair:** Fasting activates "autophagy" — your body cleans damaged cells, improving health and slowing aging.
- **Simplicity:** No complex meal plans. You just follow a timing window.

Popular Fasting Windows (Choose What Fits You)

1. **12:12 Method (Beginner-friendly)**
   - 12 hours eating window, 12 hours fasting.
   - Example: Breakfast at 8 am → Dinner by 8 pm.
2. **14:10 Method (Most Popular for Women)**
   - 10-hour eating window, 14-hour fasting.
   - Example: Eat between 10 am and 8 pm.
3. **16:8 Method (Advanced)**
   - 8-hour eating window, 16-hour fasting.
   - Example: Eat between 12 pm and 8 pm (skip breakfast).

For married women, **14:10** works best. It's flexible, family-friendly, and sustainable.

What to Eat During Eating Window

- Balanced meals (refer to Chapter 4).
- High protein + fiber = fewer cravings.
- Avoid overeating just because "time is limited."

Remember: Fasting is about **when you eat**, not eating twice the amount.

What to Drink During Fasting Window

- Water (plain or infused with lemon/jeera).
- Green tea / black tea (no sugar, no milk).
- Black coffee (optional).
- Herbal teas (tulsi, chamomile).

Avoid: milk, juice, biscuits, or even "a little snack." Anything with calories breaks the fast.

Tips to Succeed with Intermittent Fasting

1. **Start Slow:** Begin with 12:12, then move to 14:10.
2. **Stay Hydrated:** Often hunger is just thirst.
3. **Plan Dinner Early:** Helps extend your fast naturally overnight.
4. **Don't Overthink Breakfast:** Replace it with water, tea, or coffee.
5. **Listen to Your Body:** If you feel dizzy, eat something light. IF should heal, not harm.

A Sample Day (14:10 Window)

- **7:30 am:** Warm water + walk/stretch.
- **10:00 am:** First meal (paneer upma + green tea).
- **2:00 pm:** Lunch (dal, sabji, roti, curd).
- **6:00 pm:** Snack (nuts + fruit).
- **7:30 pm:** Dinner (dal soup + vegetables).
- **8:00 pm → 10:00 am:** Fasting window (only water/tea).

✦ The Key Insight:

Intermittent fasting is not a diet. It's a **pattern of eating** that gives your body time to heal, balance hormones, and burn fat naturally.

When done right, it fits beautifully into an Indian married woman's lifestyle — especially if you keep dinners early and light.

Chapter 10

SUPPLEMENTS & PROTEIN POWDERS

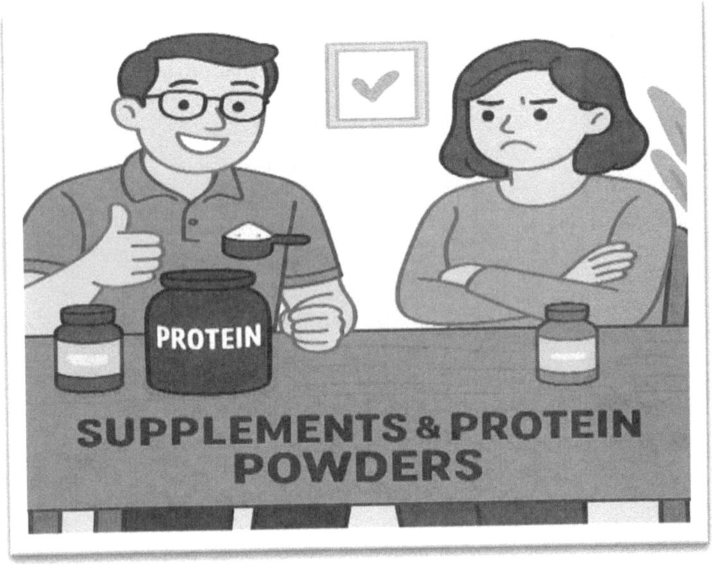

Walk into any pharmacy or open Instagram, and you'll be bombarded with ads: "This powder melts fat," "These capsules block carbs," "Drink this shake, lose 10 kg in 10 days."

No wonder most women feel confused. Do you really need supplements? Are protein powders safe? Or are they just another money-making scam?

The truth is: **most supplements are unnecessary** if your diet is balanced. But a few — the right ones — can make your fat-loss journey easier, safer, and faster.

1. Protein Powders – Friend or Foe?

Most Indian diets are **too low in protein.** (Rice, chapati, idli, dosa = carbs. Very little protein.)
Low protein = slow metabolism, muscle loss, more cravings.

That's why **protein powders** can be a convenient option.

✅**Safe Choices:**

- Whey protein (best quality, from milk).
- Plant-based protein (pea, soy, brown rice) – good for vegetarians.

❌**Avoid:**

- Cheap powders with added sugar, flavors, or steroids.
- Weight-gain shakes (loaded with sugar).

How to Use:

- 1 scoop (20–25g protein) after workout or as a breakfast smoothie.
- Mix with water, not milk (less calories, easier digestion).

- Not compulsory — if you can eat eggs, paneer, dal, chicken, or fish regularly, you may not need it.

2. Vitamins & Minerals – The Essentials

Modern diets + stress = hidden deficiencies. The most common ones in married women are:

- **Vitamin D:** Deficiency → tiredness, bone pain, low mood.
  Supplement: 1000–2000 IU daily (check blood test).
- **Vitamin B12:** Deficiency → fatigue, brain fog.
  Supplement: B12 tablets or injections (if vegetarian, more important).
- **Iron:** Deficiency → hair fall, weakness (common after childbirth).

Supplement: Only if blood test shows low levels.

3. Omega-3 (Fish Oil / Flaxseed Oil)

- Good for heart, brain, and reducing inflammation.
- Helps with fat metabolism and mood balance.

Especially useful if your diet is low in fish.

4. Calcium & Magnesium

- Crucial for bone strength (women lose bone density after 30).
- Magnesium also improves sleep and reduces stress eating.

5. Supplements You Don't Need

- "Fat burners" → Mostly caffeine + harmful stimulants.
- "Detox teas" → Just laxatives, temporary water loss.
- "Slimming pills" → Dangerous side effects, not sustainable.

A Simple Supplement Starter Kit (for Most Women)

1. **Vitamin D** (daily or weekly as prescribed).
2. **Omega-3** (fish oil capsule or flaxseed oil).
3. **Protein Powder** (optional, if diet protein is low).
4. **Multivitamin** (general coverage if diet is irregular).

Always check with your doctor before starting — especially if you're on medicines or pregnant.

✦ The Key Insight:

Supplements are not magic bullets. They can **support** your journey but cannot **replace real food, exercise, and sleep.**

Think of them as the **supporting actors**, not the hero. The hero is still *your lifestyle.*

Chapter 11

SAUNA, COLD SHOWERS & DETOX MYTHS

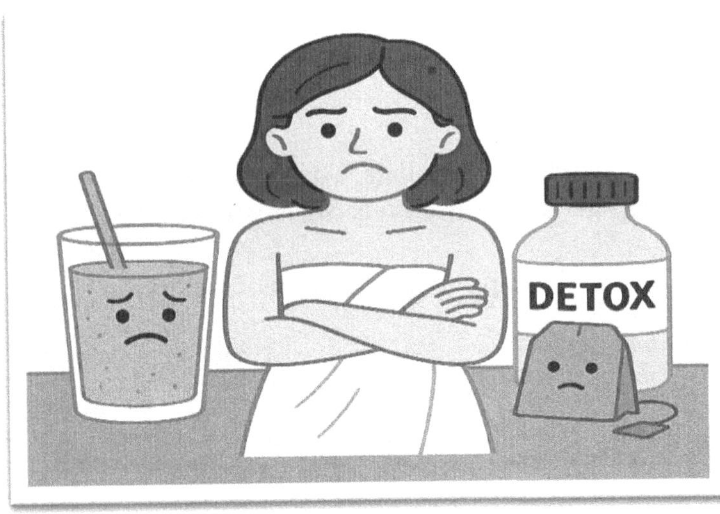

The word *"detox"* is everywhere. Instagram, YouTube, diet ads — all promising quick weight loss through sweat rooms, juice cleanses, or ice-cold showers. But here's the truth: **your body already has a natural detox system.** It's called your **liver, kidneys, lungs, and skin.**

Let's break down the most popular "detox fads" and what science actually says.

1. Saunas – Sweating Out Toxins?

Sitting in a sauna does make you sweat a lot. You feel lighter, even slimmer for a short while. But:

- Most of that "weight loss" is just **water loss**, not fat loss.
- Sweating does not remove toxins — your **liver and kidneys** do that job.
- Saunas are good for relaxation, improved circulation, and muscle recovery, but they don't "burn fat."

Verdict: Use saunas for relaxation, not as a weight-loss tool.

2. Cold Showers – Do They Burn Fat?

Cold showers have become trendy, with claims that they "activate brown fat" and boost metabolism. Here's the truth:

- Cold exposure can slightly activate brown fat (a fat type that burns calories for heat).
- But the effect is **tiny** — a few extra calories, not kilos.
- The real benefit is **mental refreshment** — it improves mood, reduces stress, and wakes you up.

Verdict: Great for energy and stress relief, but not a fat-loss miracle.

3. Juice Cleanses & Detox Drinks

Ads often promise: *"Drink this green juice for 7 days, melt belly fat!"*
Reality check:

- Juices remove fiber → sugar spikes → cravings.
- You lose some weight quickly, but it's mostly **water and muscle**, not fat.
- Long cleanses can even **slow metabolism** and cause nutrient deficiencies.

Verdict: Fresh juices are fine as part of a meal, but detox diets are unsustainable and harmful if prolonged.

4. The Real Detox: Your Body's Natural System

Instead of expensive cleanses, support your body's natural detox organs:

- **Liver:** Protected by eating less sugar, alcohol, and processed food.
- **Kidneys:** Supported by drinking enough water.
- **Lungs:** Helped by exercise and avoiding smoke/pollution.
- **Skin:** Cleansed by hydration and sweating during normal workouts.

What Actually Works (The Real Detox Routine)

✅ Drink 2–3 liters of water daily.
✅ Eat more vegetables (fiber helps remove waste).
✅ Sleep 7–8 hours (body repairs itself at night).
✅ Exercise daily (improves circulation & natural detox).
✅ Cut sugar, junk food, and alcohol (burden on liver).

✦ The Key Insight:

You don't need fancy detox teas, sweat rooms, or ice baths to "cleanse" your body. Your body already has a detox system. What it needs is **support, not shortcuts.**

CHAPTER 12

HOW TO STAY ON TRACK WHEN LIFE GETS BUSY

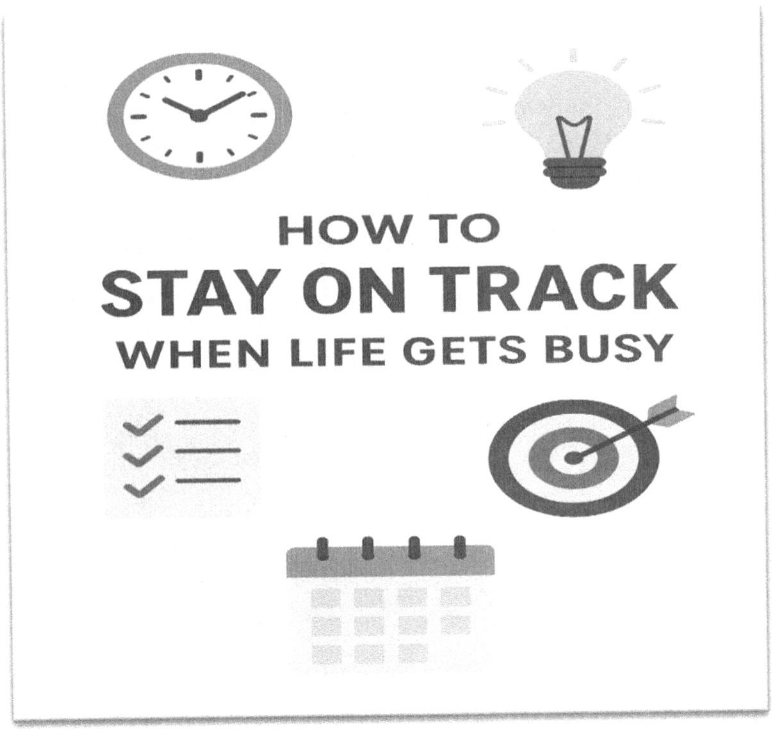

Let's be honest: life after marriage is never smooth. Work deadlines, kids' exams, in-laws visiting, weddings, festivals, travel — every week brings something new.

This is when most women slip. *"I'll start again next week..."* becomes a cycle. But here's the truth: **you don't need perfection to lose weight. You just need consistency.** Even on the busiest days, you can stay on track with smart strategies.

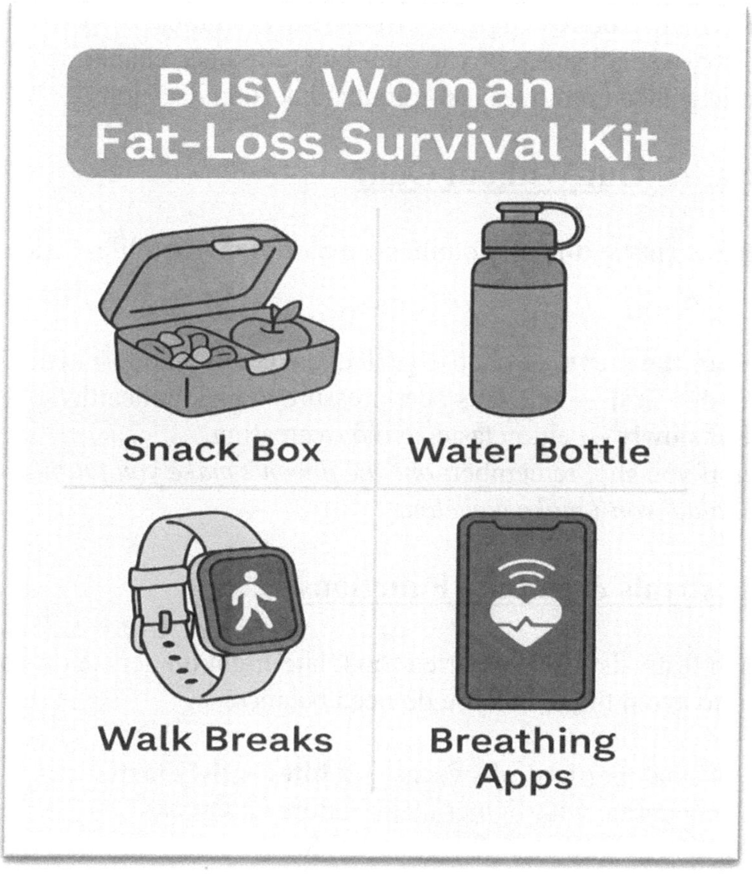
Busy Woman
Fat-Loss Survival Kit
Snack Box
Water Bottle
Walk Breaks
Breathing
Apps

1. The 80/20 Rule

- Eat healthy **80% of the time**, and allow 20% flexibility.
- Example: If you eat 15 meals in a week, 12 should be clean, 3 can be relaxed.

This way, you stay consistent without feeling deprived.

2. Plan Ahead (Meal Prepping Saves You)

- Cook extra dal, sabji, or grilled chicken → store in fridge.
- Keep nuts, boiled eggs, and fruits ready to grab.
- Carry a small snack box in your bag (almonds, chana).

Planning ahead removes last-minute junk food decisions.

3. Eating Out Without Guilt

Social events and family outings are part of married life. Instead of stressing:

- **Scan the menu** → choose grilled, baked, or tandoori items.
- **Order first** → prevents peer pressure to pick unhealthy.
- **Eat slowly** → enjoy taste, avoid overeating.

Even if you slip, remember: *one meal won't make you fat, just like one salad won't make you slim.*

4. Festivals & Family Functions

Indian festivals = sweets, fried food, late-night dinners. You don't need to avoid them, but you do need balance.

- Eat small portions of sweets — **2 bites satisfy taste**.
- Compensate with lighter meals before and after.
- Focus on family bonding, not just food.

5. Work Travel & Holidays

Travel often derails routines. Stay prepared:

- Carry protein bars, nuts, or roasted chana.
- Drink water before meals to avoid overeating.
- Walk whenever possible — airports, sightseeing, hotel corridors.

Vacations are to relax, not relapse.

6. Stress & Emotional Eating

When life gets stressful, food becomes comfort. But stress-eating doesn't solve problems — it only adds guilt.

- Replace food with **quick stress relief rituals:** 5 deep breaths, 10-min walk, journaling, or calming tea.
- If you must snack, choose **protein + fiber** (nuts, yogurt, fruit) instead of sugar.

7. Quick Workouts on Busy Days

Even 10 minutes is enough when life gets hectic.

- 20 squats + 10 push-ups + 20 step-ups + 20-sec plank.
  Done! A mini workout keeps your metabolism active.

✦ The Key Insight:

Success is not about being perfect every day. It's about **never quitting, even on the busiest days.** Small, smart decisions add up to big results.

Remember: The women who succeed are not the ones who never fall — they're the ones who always get back up.

CHAPTER 13

REIGNITE CONFIDENCE & BODY IMAGE AFTER MARRIAGE

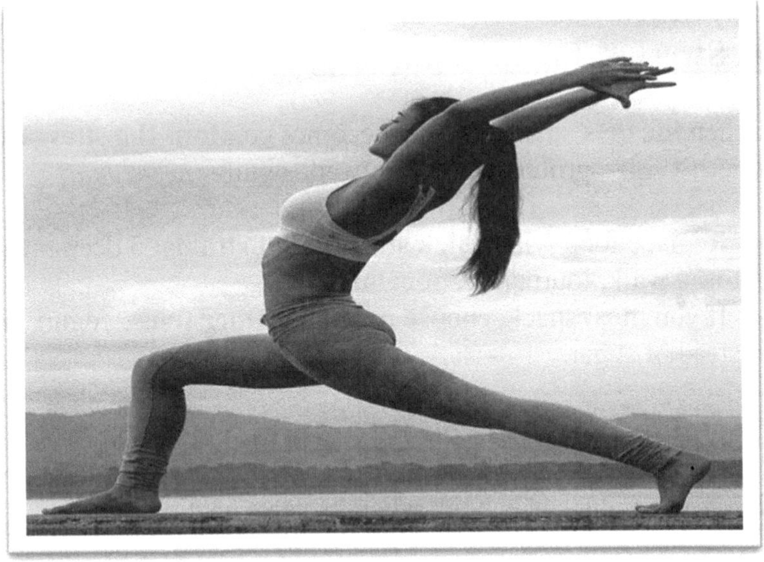

Marriage changes a woman's life in beautiful ways — but it also often changes how she sees herself.

Between juggling responsibilities, taking care of everyone else, and dealing with subtle comments from society (*"You've put on weight after marriage,"* or *"Why don't you look like you used to?"*), many women slowly lose touch with the confident, radiant version of themselves.

This chapter is about helping you **find her again.**

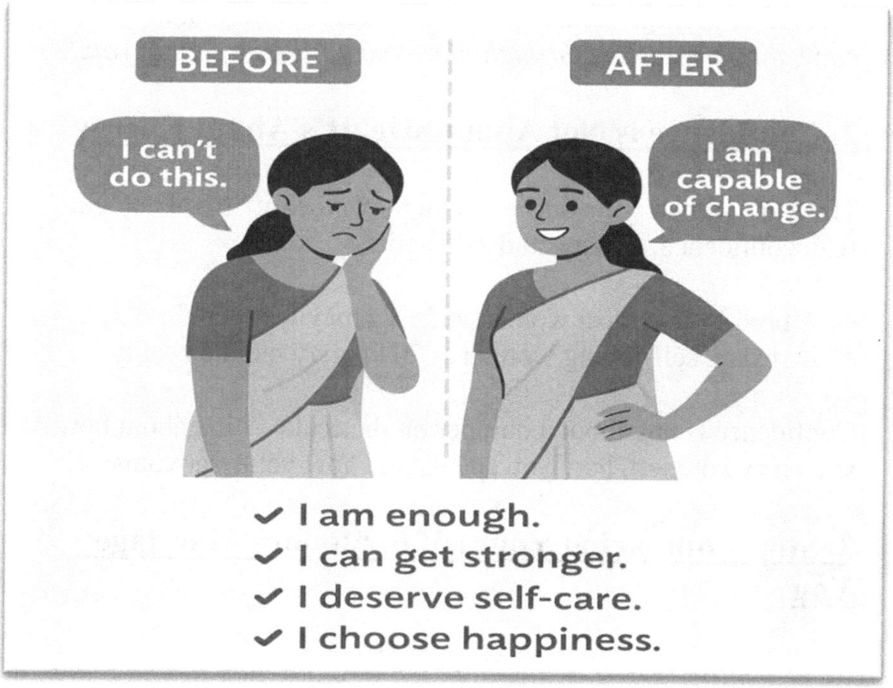
BEFORE
AFTER
I can't do this.
I am capable of change.
✔ I am enough.
✔ I can get stronger.
✔ I deserve self-care.
✔ I choose happiness.

1. Stop Seeing Your Body as the Enemy

Too many women stare into the mirror and only notice flaws:

- "My tummy is bigger."
- "My arms look fat."
- "I don't look like I used to before marriage."

The truth is: **your body is not your enemy.**
It's carried you through love, stress, work, pregnancy, family life. It deserves respect, not punishment.

Instead of saying: *"I hate my belly,"* start saying: *"Thank you, body, for carrying me through life — now I'll take care of you."*

2. Confidence is Not About Size, It's About Energy

Think of women you admire — are they all slim? No. They glow with confidence, energy, and self-belief.

- A tired, self-critical woman at 55 kg may feel "fat."
- A strong, self-loving woman at 70 kg may radiate beauty.

Confidence is not about a number on the scale — it's about how you carry yourself, how you speak, and how you treat yourself.

3. Stop Comparing Yourself to "Before Marriage" You

Many women say: *"I just want to look like I did before marriage."* But life changes. Your body has adapted, your hormones have shifted, you've taken on responsibilities.

The goal is not to "go back." The goal is to **create a new, stronger version of you now.**

4. Small Habits That Build Confidence Daily

- **Dress for yourself:** Wear clothes that make you feel good today, not after you lose weight.
- **Move with pride:** Walk tall, shoulders back, chin up. Posture alone changes how people see you.
- **Celebrate progress:** Lost 1 kg? Clothes fitting better? More energy? Write it down.
- **Self-care rituals:** Skincare, hair care, meditation, even 10 minutes of silence — all remind you that *you matter too.*

5. Speak Kindly to Yourself

Your inner dialogue shapes your confidence. Instead of:
❌"I'll never lose weight."
❌"I look terrible."
Say:
✅"I'm improving every day."
✅"I am more than my weight — I am strong, smart, and valuable."

Talk to yourself the way you would talk to your best friend.

✦ The Key Insight:

Confidence and body image are not rewards you get *after* losing weight. They are tools you use *during* the journey. The more you respect your body now, the faster it will transform.

Chapter 14

MENTAL HEALTH, BODY IMAGE & DEPRESSION

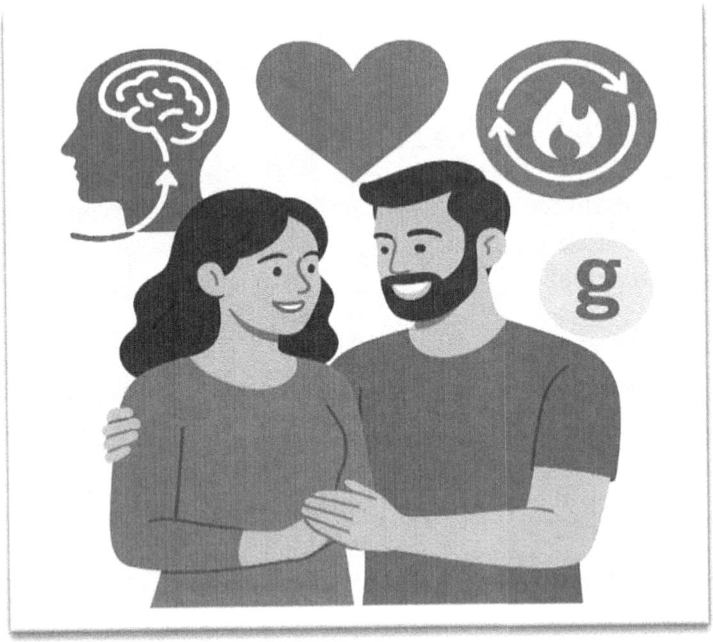

Behind every extra kilo, there is often more than just food. There are unspoken emotions:

- Stress from juggling family and work.
- Pressure from in-laws or society.
- Loneliness in marriage, even when surrounded by people.
- A quiet sadness that food temporarily soothes.

This is why weight loss is not just about calories and workouts — it's also about **mental health.**

1. Stress and Cortisol – The Silent Weight Gainer

When you're under constant stress, your body produces **cortisol** (the stress hormone).

- Cortisol increases cravings for sugary, fried, and comfort foods.
- It signals the body to store more fat around the belly.
- Even if you eat less, stress can block fat loss.

This is why some women say: *"I'm dieting, but nothing is working."* Stress is sabotaging them silently.

2. Emotional Eating – Food as Comfort

Food becomes more than food when you're sad, bored, or overwhelmed. A packet of chips or a sweet feels like a "hug" — but only for a few minutes. After that comes guilt, shame, and self-blame.

Breaking the cycle:

- Before eating, ask: *"Am I hungry or just stressed?"*
- Replace food with a **comfort ritual** → journaling, walking, calling a friend, sipping herbal tea.

- If you must eat, choose **protein + fiber snacks** (nuts, fruit + yogurt) instead of sugar.

3. Depression and Weight

Depression and weight gain often feed each other:

- Low mood → overeating → weight gain → lower self-esteem → deeper depression.
- Some antidepressant medications can also cause weight gain.

Solutions:

- Seek professional help without shame. Mental health is as real as physical health.
- Add movement — exercise releases endorphins (natural antidepressants).
- Practice gratitude journaling — write 3 things you're thankful for daily.

4. Body Image Pressure after Marriage

Society is often cruel. A newly married woman is expected to look slim, glowing, and perfect. Comments like *"You've gained after marriage"* or *"You don't look like before"* can hurt deeply.

How to protect your self-image:

- Remember: people's comments reflect their mindset, not your worth.
- Focus on your health, not their opinion.
- Surround yourself with supportive voices — a friend, spouse, or even online community.

5. Simple Mental Health Habits That Heal

- **Sleep 7–8 hours** → lack of sleep worsens stress hormones.
- **Deep breathing (5 minutes daily)** → lowers cortisol instantly.
- **Daily sunlight** → boosts Vitamin D and mood.
- **Movement = Medicine** → even a 20-min walk lifts depression.
- **Say NO without guilt** → protect your boundaries, reduce overwhelm.

🠗 The Key Insight:

Weight loss is not only about what you eat — it's about what you feel. Heal your mind, and your body will follow. Stress, emotional eating, and depression are not weaknesses. They are signals from your body asking you to slow down, care, and heal.

Chapter 15

LONG-TERM FAT LOSS— HOW TO MAINTAIN RESULTS FOR LIFE

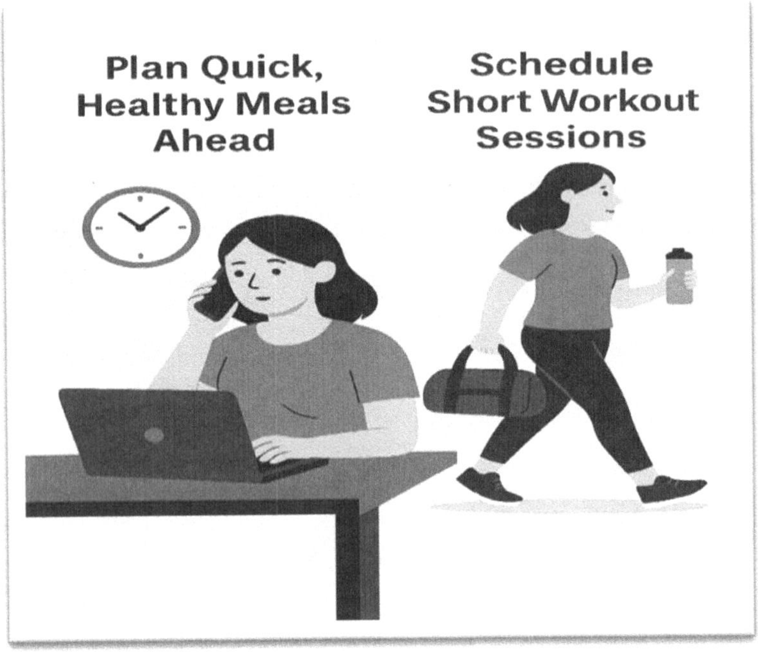

Losing weight is exciting. But let's be honest — keeping it off is the real challenge.

How many women do you know who tried a diet, lost weight, and then regained it all (sometimes even more)? This is called **yo-yo dieting** — and it's both frustrating and unhealthy.

The good news? **Permanent fat loss is possible.** You just need the right mindset, habits, and systems.

1. Shift Your Goal: From "Diet" to "Lifestyle"

Diets have start and end dates. Lifestyles don't.

- A "diet" mindset says: *"I'll eat clean until I lose 5 kg."*
- A "lifestyle" mindset says: *"I'll eat healthy because I want energy, confidence, and long-term health."*

Ask yourself: *"Can I do this for the next 5 years?"* If not, it's not sustainable.

2. Build Non-Negotiable Habits

Permanent fat loss is about small habits you repeat forever.

- **Daily movement:** 20–30 min walk/workout.
- **Protein in every meal:** Keeps metabolism strong.
- **Dinner before 8 pm:** Simple, powerful rule.
- **Sleep by 10:30 pm:** Protects hormones.
- **Hydrate:** 2–3 liters water daily.

These become part of your identity, not just a "weight-loss phase."

3. Watch Out for the "Comfort Trap"

After losing weight, many women relax:

- They go back to old eating patterns.
- Exercise becomes irregular.
- Cheat days turn into cheat weeks.

Solution: **Maintenance Plan**

- Keep weighing yourself weekly (not obsessively, just check-in).
- Have a "reset routine" (like the 10-Day Reset in Chapter 8) whenever you slip.
- Stay active even on holidays.

4. Keep Evolving

Your body changes with age, hormones, pregnancy, and menopause. What worked at 30 may not work at 40.

Stay flexible. Learn, adjust, and adapt. Fat loss is a journey, not a one-time event.

5. Protect Your Environment

- Keep healthy foods stocked → If junk is not in the house, you won't eat it.
- Surround yourself with people who support your journey.
- Avoid toxic "diet culture" voices that shame you.

6. Celebrate Non-Scale Victories

The weighing scale is only one measure. Confidence, glowing skin, better sleep, fitting into old clothes — these matter more.

Focus on becoming the **healthiest version of yourself**, not the skinniest.

The Key Insight:

Long-term fat loss is not about being perfect every day. It's about building a life where **healthy living feels normal.** Once your lifestyle supports your health, weight becomes easy to maintain.

Chapter 16

PLANNING GUILT-FREE VACATIONS & CHEAT DAYS

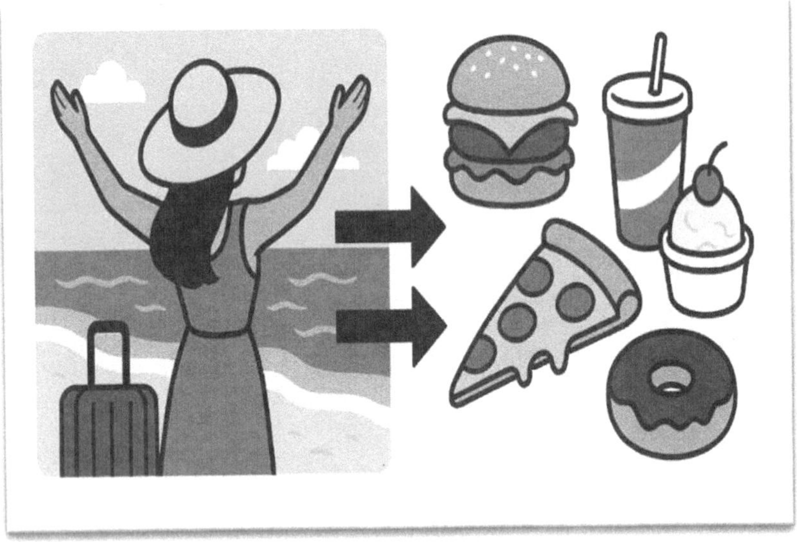

Food is more than calories. It's love, celebration, culture, and memories. Marriage brings weddings, birthdays, festivals, vacations, and family functions — and avoiding them is impossible (and unhealthy for the heart).

The secret is not to avoid these moments, but to enjoy them **without guilt** while staying on track.

1. Redefine "Cheat Day"

Most women think: *"Cheat day means eat anything, everything!"* That mindset often undoes a whole week's progress.

Instead, think **"Treat Meal."**

- One meal where you enjoy your favorite food guilt-free.
- Portion control matters — one slice of cake, not half the cake.
- Enjoy slowly, with family, without shame.

Remember: **One treat meal won't make you fat, just like one salad won't make you slim.**

2. Parties & Weddings – The Survival Guide

- **Eat before you go:** A small protein snack (boiled eggs, paneer, nuts) prevents overeating.
- **Start with salad & protein:** Fill half your plate with healthy choices first.
- **Taste, don't binge:** Take small portions of favorite dishes, enjoy every bite.
- **Drink smart:** Skip sugary drinks; stick to water, lime soda, or one small glass of wine (if you drink).

3. Festivals & Family Functions

In India, festivals = sweets, fried foods, endless meals.
The balance strategy:

- Enjoy **2–3 bites** of sweets instead of 2–3 pieces.
- Compensate by eating light before and after.
- Remember: festivals are about **people, rituals, joy** — not just food.

4. Vacations & Holidays – Travel Smart

Vacations are not for dieting — they're for living! But you can stay in control:

- **80/20 rule:** Eat healthy for 2 meals, enjoy freedom in 1 meal.
- **Walk more:** Sightseeing, beaches, or exploring streets = natural exercise.
- **Pack smart snacks:** Nuts, protein bars, roasted chana — saves you from random junk.
- **Hydrate:** Carry a water bottle everywhere.

Trick: If you gain 1–2 kg during vacation, don't panic. It's usually water weight and will settle with your normal routine.

5. Bounce Back After Indulgence

The real danger is not one party or trip — it's the guilt that follows. Women say: *"I've spoiled everything, now what's the point?"* and give up.

Solution:

- Next meal → go back to healthy eating. Don't "punish" with starvation.
- Add 15 extra minutes of walking the next day.
- Drink more water, sleep well.

Weight gain from one event is temporary. Weight gain from guilt and giving up is permanent.

6. The Mindset Shift

Food is not the enemy. It's a part of life. By learning balance, you free yourself from food guilt forever.

Think of it this way: **You are not dieting, you are living.**

- 80% health, 20% enjoyment = lifelong success.
- No shame, no punishment, no all-or-nothing.

The Key Insight:

Vacations, parties, and celebrations are not interruptions to your journey — they're part of your journey. When you learn balance, you can be slim, confident, and free **while still enjoying life to the fullest.**

Chapter 17

LIFESTYLE BLUEPRINTS– PICK YOUR PATH

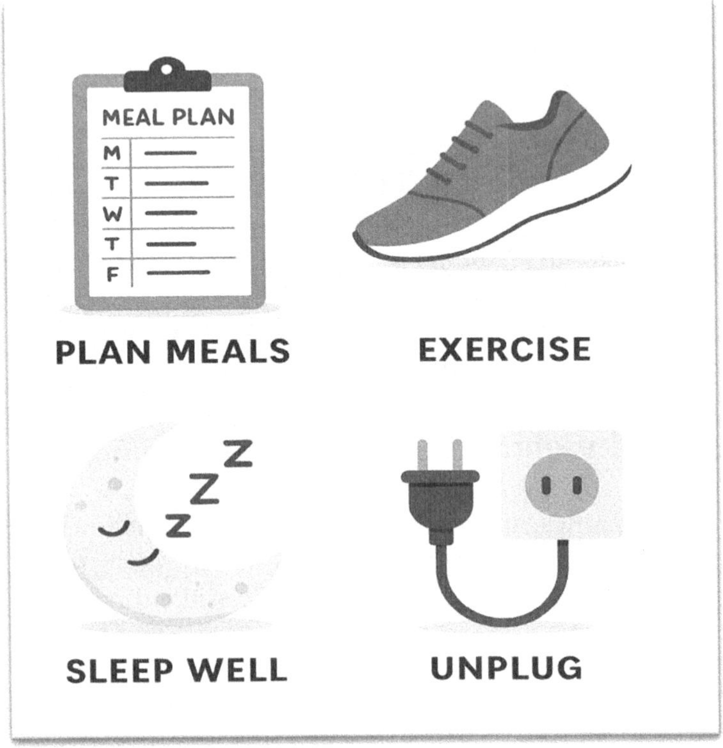

Every woman's life is different. Some are full-time professionals, some manage home and family, some are young newlyweds, others are mothers juggling kids and work.

That's why you don't need "the perfect plan" — you need **your perfect plan.**

Here are 4 ready-made blueprints you can adapt to your life.

1. The Working Professional Blueprint

For women balancing office, commute, and home.

- **Morning:** Warm water + lemon, 10 min stretching.
- **Breakfast (office-friendly):** Overnight oats with nuts, or protein smoothie.
- **Lunch (packed):** Chapati + dal + sabji + salad.
- **Snack (office desk):** Nuts + fruit, green tea.
- **Dinner (after office):** Grilled paneer/chicken/fish + salad.
- **Workout:** 20 min brisk walk after work, or short home workout.

Key Tip: Carry smart snacks to avoid office junk food.

2. The Homemaker Blueprint

For women managing housework, cooking, and family routines.

- **Morning:** Herbal tea + 20 min yoga/walk before household work.
- **Breakfast:** 2 boiled eggs / sprouts upma + chutney.
- **Lunch:** Millet/roti + dal + sabji + curd.
- **Snack:** Roasted chana + buttermilk.
- **Dinner (with family):** Soup + stir-fried vegetables.
- **Extra Movement:** Take stairs, 10-min walk after meals.

Key Tip: Use the family's food but adjust portions (½ rice, more veggies/protein).

3. The Young Married Woman Blueprint

For newlyweds adjusting to family expectations & social life.

- **Morning:** Warm water + light stretching.
- **Breakfast:** Paneer paratha (less oil) + curd.
- **Lunch:** Normal family meal (control portions, double veggies).
- **Snack (with spouse/friends):** Choose fruit plate / nuts instead of fried snacks.
- **Dinner (early):** Dal soup or grilled dish + salad.
- **Workout:** Couple walk after dinner or short HIIT session at home.

Key Tip: Don't fight family food traditions — learn smart swaps and portion control.

4. The Busy Mother Blueprint

For women balancing children, school runs, and little time for self-care.

- **Morning:** Quick lemon water, 10 min yoga/stretch while kids get ready.
- **Breakfast:** Boiled eggs + fruit OR smoothie (blend milk, banana, protein powder).
- **Lunch (with kids):** Rice/chapati + dal + sabji + curd. (Eat same as kids, just smaller carbs, more protein).
- **Snack:** Handful of nuts, protein bar, or fruit on the go.
- **Dinner:** One-pot meal (dal soup, khichdi with veggies, or grilled chicken with sautéed veggies).
- **Workout:** 15 min "snack workout" while kids nap/play (squats, push-ups, plank).

Key Tip: Use **mini workouts** and healthy one-pot meals to save time.

5. The Festival/Travel Blueprint (Special Situations)

For when life is not routine.

- **Before party/travel:** Eat light protein snack at home.
- **During:** Enjoy favorites in small portions.
- **After:** Drink more water, sleep well, walk extra 15 min next day.

Key Tip: Festivals & travel are temporary — get back to routine quickly.

The Key Insight:

There is no "one perfect diet." The perfect plan is the one you can follow in *your* life. Pick your blueprint, stick to it, and remember — **consistency beats perfection.**

Final Chapter

YOU DIDN'T JUST LOSE WEIGHT — YOU TOOK YOUR POWER BACK

This journey wasn't just about fat loss.

Losing weight was never just about fitting into smaller clothes. It was never only about the number on the scale.

This journey was about something much bigger.

It was about proving to yourself that you are **stronger than excuses.**
It was about saying "no" to the voices that told you, *"You can't."*
It was about choosing health over guilt, confidence over shame, and joy over fear.

You Reclaimed More Than a Body

- When you said no to junk food, you weren't just cutting calories — you were **saying yes to self-respect.**
- When you woke up early to move your body, you weren't just burning fat — you were **building discipline.**
- When you handled festivals, vacations, and stress without losing control, you weren't just avoiding weight gain — you were **proving your power.**

Every step, every choice, every struggle was not just about fat loss. It was about **taking back control of your life.**

A New You — Stronger, Braver, Happier

Now you stand at a new beginning.

- You have the strength to set boundaries.
- The confidence to look in the mirror and smile.
- The energy to live, love, and dream bigger.

This transformation is not temporary — it's a rebirth.

The Ripple Effect

When you change, the world around you changes.

- Your family sees your strength and feels inspired.
- Your children grow up watching health, not excuses.
- Your spouse feels your renewed confidence and joy.

Your journey has created ripples that will impact generations.

The Final Insight:
You didn't just lose weight. You lost fear. You lost doubt. You lost the idea that you are not enough.

And in return, you gained power. You gained freedom. You gained yourself.

Closing Note:
Every time you feel tempted to quit, remember this: **you have already proven you can rise.**

This is not the end of your journey — it is the beginning of the life you always deserved.

Walk tall. Smile wide. Live free.

Because you didn't just lose weight — **you took your power back.**

Conclusion – Your New Life Begins

Dear Reader,

If you've come this far, it means something inside you has awakened. You didn't just read another book — you began a journey of self-respect, self-care, and self-love.

You now know the truth:

- Weight gain after marriage is not your fate.
- Your hormones, your habits, and your mindset are in your control.
- Small, consistent steps create massive transformation.

This is not about dieting. This is not about punishment. This is about **choosing a life where health and happiness are your new normal.**

Your Next Step

Don't wait for "Monday" or "next month." Start today.

- Drink your water.
- Move your body for 20 minutes.
- Eat one balanced plate of food.
- Say one kind thing to yourself.

That's all it takes to keep your power alive — small wins, every single day.

Stay Connected, Stay Inspired

Transformation is easier when you're not alone.

- Share your journey with your family — let them cheer you on.
- Inspire other women — your story could save someone else's confidence.
- Connect with me on my health platforms, where I share daily guidance, tips, and motivation for women just like you.

You are part of a community now — a sisterhood of women reclaiming their power.

Final Words:

This is your time. Your season. Your rebirth.

Every morning, when you wake up, remind yourself:
"I am stronger than yesterday. My body is my ally. My health is my power."

Go live boldly, love deeply, and walk proudly. Because from this moment on…

Your new life begins.